This is an autobiographical book

Copyright © 2020 Mathieu Desormeaux
GOT ASPERGER'S?

All rights reserved
Published by Sami Desormeaux
https://www.theofficialsami.com

Edited by Sami Desormeaux & Dr. Akel Kahera
Cover by Marianne Long & Sami Desormeaux
Islamic leaf design by Sami Desormeaux

With Thanks to Jules Bss, Drahomír Posteby-Mach, Kiki Falconer, my wife and myself, Jr. Korpa, Nicola POWYS, Robert Collins, Jeremy Bishop, Greg Rakozy, Caleb Jones for the Images With Modifications and Touchups by Sami Desormeaux

This book is not intended as a substitute for the medical advice of physicians. The reader should regularly consult a trained expert in matters relating to his/her health and particularly with respect to the diagnosis of autism spectrum disorder.

Copyright Registration Number:
1171706
Canadian ISBN:
978-1-7770420-2-8

Canadian Intellectual Property Office:
Place du Portage I
50 Victoria Street
Gatineau, QC, Canada
K1A 0C9

First Canadian Edition: July 2020
Digitally uploaded in Canada

Grand-maman, in honour of your passing eleven years ago, may you be proud of your grand-children. Je t'aime!

Got Asperger's?

Sami

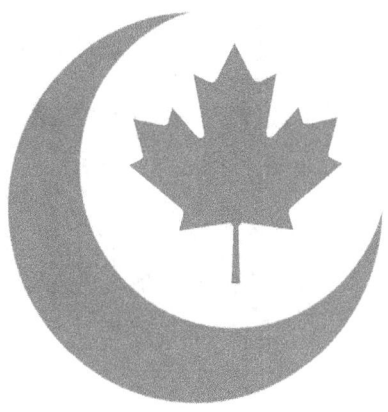

Dedicated to my long time deceased uncle Jean-Pierre Brunet and my cousin René Robert, both of whom were/are autistic

Most importantly, dedicated to my mother who only hoped her children never had to suffer from autism. Released on her birthday as a gift to her. Bonne fête m'man! Je t'aime!

With thanks to Dr. Akel Kahera for his help in editing this work

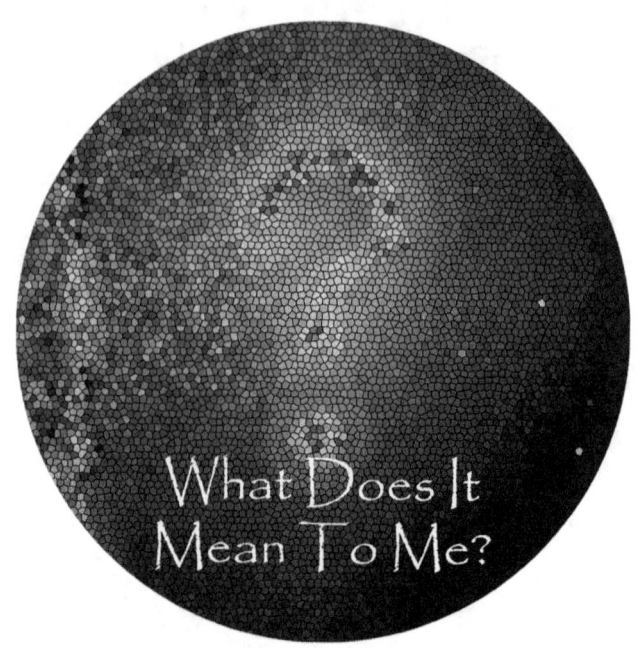

What Does It Mean To Me?

Don't let things you don't understand or have little knowledge about fool you. I have faced some struggles during my lifetime but have persevered for as long as I could thus far. If we start from the beginning, perhaps I could list my disadvantages to give you an idea of the person I am.

I was born deaf but was operated on so I could hear. My feet are flat and have a deviated bone structure in my legs due to this (not that you could really tell unless you're looking for that. For all intent and purposes, I look normal). My sister, supposedly, broke my nose and it's been crooked ever since. As you might have guessed, breathing is difficult at times. As if this wasn't enough, I have had glasses since I was eight years old.

Aside from those physical ailments, I have Asperger's, I suffer from anxiety day in and day out and I also have to live in a neurotypical world that doesn't always understand why I say the things I say, nor the things I do. Just to be clear, I have Asperger's, I do not suffer from Asperger's.

Regardless of all those annoyances and frustrations in my life, there are plenty of examples of things that have gone my way (not that Asperger's is bad). I am an extremely intelligent person, with an above average IQ, I was the first of my siblings to obtain a University Degree as well as having two published books to my name (excluding this one) at the time of writing this. On top of that, I have the knack of seeing through people and knowing who they are.

Here is the question of: What does Asperger's mean for me? Honestly? I don't know. I don't see myself as different from the world. Rather, I see the world as different. I am the norm, not the other way around. For the most part, I agree with a lot of society's tenets. I, however, don't always understand why people do things, especially harmful things they do to themselves. The body is not a temple, but it doesn't mean it should be treated like decrepit ruins.

Back to the original question of what it means, Asperger's is not part of who I am. It is who I am. Seeing the world around me, it can be quite challenging witnessing a world void of understanding. Alas, people may often judge what they don't understand and would see it as a handicap. It's not, and it never will be. How could the person you are be considered a handicap? A handicap is something which prevents you from accomplishing what you normally do or would like to do.

Those of us with Asperger's tend to be extremely creative. What I do is use this creativity to fuel my talent. Others have diverse talents, including painting, music, acting or even drawing. We tend to focus on something very specific. I may not be that great when it comes to other things, but having a single focus is amazing.

Personally, for example, I have the ability to write a love letter within ten minutes. While most people would struggle and spend days, I don't need that much time. It's a craft to be sure, but not one I struggle with. I suppose to answer the original question, that's what it means to me. Asperger's has given me a talent I can use for different purposes, including writing for others, myself, or my wife.

When I see others agonizing over words, they wish to convey to their loved one, it perplexes me. Then again, since it comes easily to me, I can't expect others to have that same ease I do concerning this.

I also have a knack for editing other people's work, as my brain understands what to modify to make it more interesting or less redundant. Mind you, sometimes redundancy can be effective if used correctly. Otherwise, it can be messy.

I remember back in the day when GameSpy was around. It was a gaming software with different games on it. I would play this writing game where you had to write something specific about a certain topic if I recall correctly, within a limited time frame. Probably something like five or ten minutes, and the other players would vote on who wrote the best paragraph. I won all the time. I used humour and deep-seated sadness to win.

For me, when I see creativity around, it amazes me to no end. Of course, I am only referring to something I find interesting. I have no interest in seeing a portrait of flowers for example. On the other hand, if you can demonstrate your talents with something with a sci-fi theme, I will be extremely interested.

The human brain itself is so complex, and the ability to generate masterpieces is no small feat. Imagine this: Someone was able to install an operating system on a computer; someone was able to put computer components together; someone was able to create those pieces; and finally, someone was capable of somehow managing for an operating system to work on a computer system. How is that even possible? We are amazing as a [human] race.

As a computer expert, I never have taken the time to learn how that is even possible. When you think of the power of the human brain, it takes someone special to come up with these and put them together. How does someone make words appear in a word processor? Sure, it's programmed and so on, but the behind-the-scenes part of it must be fascinating.

All of this to say that someone with Asperger's has the potential to be something most people can only dream of. Focus on a single expertise means the brain has had to be shaped by all those years of practicing the craft. That being said, it's remarkable when someone can focus on a single thing and make it his own.

Therefore, what Asperger's mean to me is a means to achieve greatness incarnate. Everyone has the ability to develop into something extraordinary, if they are willing to invest the time and effort into it. Yet for others and myself, it is a gift that requires only the time to actually perform it. It is a natural talent that cannot be explained, but by the mere fact that it is a talent which exists.

The best example I know of is an autistic man by the name of Derek Paravicini. He is a musical pianist prodigy. I have seen his mentor play a random piece, and Paravicini was able to play the exact same notes in a second. That being said, Paravicini is a musical prodigy who has the ability to play whatever he so chooses. This type of gift cannot be explained. Pure, raw talent.

How can we compare potential versus talent? There is a difference between both. The former is what you see in sports, where they evaluate rookies based on their potential to achieve greatness. As for the latter, talent cannot be measured, as it exists in a raw and pure form. How do you evaluate this? By default, since it's already good, it would simply be a matter of how good.

Unlocking your potential is a matter of training and sticking with it until you're at the top. Actual talent is where you've always been beyond unlocked potential. It exists, because it always has and always will, unless your body tells you can't anymore.

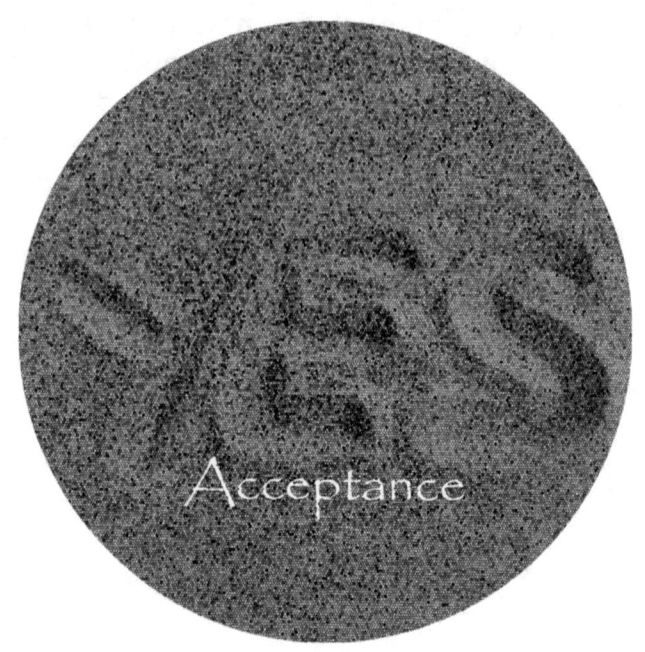

Acceptance

Having the capacity to accept yourself as you are can be difficult, depending on your personality and how willing you are to admit that part of yourself. I have seen others not caring at all and being cool with it. Even though I can't speak for the rest, that has been an extremely difficult task for me. No human being is the same, even when there are seven billion people in the world. You may look alike, act the same, or even have the same personality, but at some point, there will be a difference.

It has been enormously tough for me to deal with the person I am now, as well as having to still deal with how others are around me. I always considered it problematic to only worry about other individuals and how they were. Now, there are two things I need to look out for.

Who I am does explain a lot of things, while allowing me to understand why I feel the way I do and why I do the way I do things (which will be explained later). Yet, it has been hard to accept the person I am, because of stigmas attached to it. Since for all intent and purposes I behave the same as most people in many aspects, they don't realise I am different.

Regardless of this, I am learning to look past what others could see in me. I certainly have shortcomings, yet my qualities more than make up for what I lack in this world. Most importantly, I can't change who I am, as Asperger's is not a part of me, but it's who I am. I can't just remove that part of me like you could replace a body part.

This being said, Asperger's make me the person I am, as my brain is wired the way it is. It's not something you can change. If it was, then you would have countless people getting surgeries, going to therapy or taking medication. Your brain doesn't work that way. Unless you're trying to harm yourself on purpose (or by accident), your brain is immutable until natural degradation through time.

Since Asperger's is not a behaviour, it can't be modified. Sure, you can make compromises or do something different for your significant other, but none of that changes the person you are or the frustration that entails with having to make those changes. The person you are at the core is the person you are for the rest of your life.

As it's not a behaviour but the way your brain is wired, it has become easier for me to understand the person I am. Despite the fact that at times I have done certain things that may have irritated others or outright annoyed them, I now realise that this isn't my fault. I totally get that this doesn't help the other person feel better about the situation, but at least there's a reason for it.

This, in part, has enabled me to accept that I won't change who I am, because I neurologically simply can't. It's not a question of wanting or not wanting to change certain behaviours or patterns. I am fully aware that certain things I do aggravates some individuals, and it has proven very challenging for me to abstain from doing those things.

There still remains the question: How do you accept yourself, when many can't understand what it feels like? Imagine having an itch that keeps coming back. First on your head, then your chest and finally your legs. You scratch those parts because they itch, and then you scratch them again later because they still itch. That is what it feels like for people not to understand.

As I said earlier, because I appear the same as most individuals, no one understands why I feel the way I feel about certain situations. Due to this, it's easier to accept that the person I am is not because I'm weird or different. It's simply because of Asperger's.

With having Asperger's, there are things that come with the territory. At least for me, these are some of the things about me that wouldn't ever change: I will always take care of my wife and any children we may have; I have a well of unconditional love; I am extremely patient for the most part. As long as we have been married, I have never yelled at her.

On the other hand, I certainly do some things others may consider annoying. For example, my wife can testify that when I want attention, I am very loud about it, as I show an exuberant display of it. She calls me dramatic! When it comes to music, I need to listen to the version of the song I enjoy, otherwise I can't as it will bother me to no end. And when I want something, I want it now.

What's very ironic about this, is that I always believed this might have been because we, as a society, have learnt to want things now due to the evolution of technology. I was wrong about that. I can't help wanting things now. When I must wait, it kills me. Strangely enough, despite being very patient, I need things now. I tend to be very patient about most things except if I need my wife to look at something, I want to show her. Be it writing or something ingame (videogames).

All in all, I understand a lot more now that the reason I do things is not because of a petty or childish desire to need things a certain way. Instead, it has simply to do with the fact that my brain is wired that way due to Asperger's. It's a relief to know there's a valid reason for the way I am, and the way I do things. Including the constant use of the serial comma, like in the previous sentence. I could avoid the serial comma, but it just wouldn't make any sense to me. So, I have to use it.

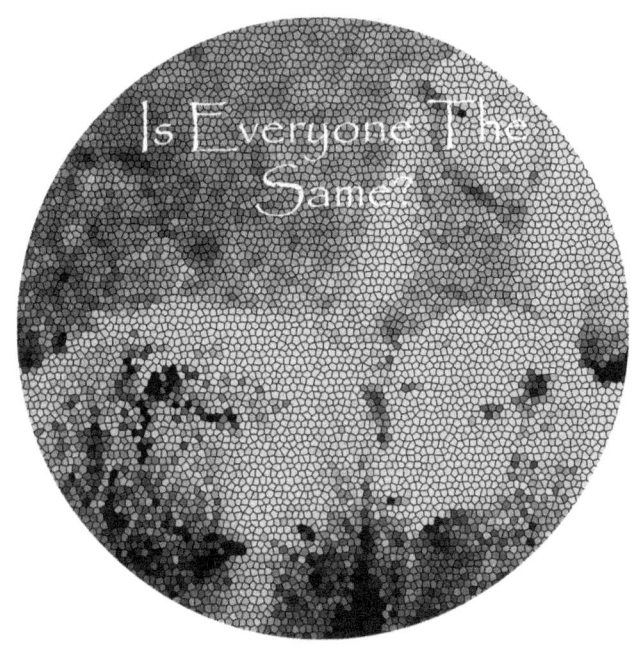

The short answer to that question is: No. The longer answer is more complicated. The reality is that everyone, to a certain extent, is the same. Then again, how do you define what that entails and how much of it is the same or different?

If we agree to live by the same rules in a society, therefore we live a similar life. At the same time, we have our own preferences, likes and dislikes. In theory, that would mean we are different, no? How can you reconcile the true answer of: Yes, we are the same, yet we are different?

Someone similar to me might find certain things just as annoying, or it may not bother them at all. They may need to have certain things a certain way, while I might need them a different way. In our uniqueness, the more things are different, the more they are the same. That is called a paradox. It makes no sense whatsoever, but it does at the same time.

You could argue this is just semantics or utter nonsense. The truth is much harder to understand. For example, we could claim that my preference for a specific movie over the one you prefer makes us different. At the same time, since we both enjoy movies, then... yeah. This is a simple paradox. It makes sense, yet it doesn't. We like movies, just not the same. Ok, but both are movies.

As we differ on several topics, we remain the same during a large chunk of our lives. The biggest difference for two neurotypicals may be something like political affiliations. For me, that would also be true. However, in terms of who your favourite basketball player is, or what movie franchise is better, that is huge. You may not care or see any reason argue about this, I would. It's not that I'd want to, but because I'd have to.

The reality is that what matters to neurotypicals are usually about more 'important' matters, while for me, what may seem trivial isn't. There is, of course, a degree of importance that most people attach to events, objects, or topics.

An easy example of this for me would include the fact that when dishes are piling up and I need to clean them, it becomes a lot easier for me if they are stacked a certain way. If they are in the sink and all over the place, without regard to a specific order, it becomes mentally difficult for me to start doing them.

Eventually I will, but it takes longer. The question at that point becomes how? Not the mechanic, but simply the 'how am I going to do this?' On top of this, when I put utensils in the dishwasher, I need to separate normal utensils together, while placing steak knives and other types of utensils separately.

While people would state that it's not that hard, they obviously don't understand. I suppose, how could they? Realistically, I couldn't expect someone else to understand. At best, they could comprehend that I deal with things differently. In terms of why those things affect me the way they do, they will never understand. Just as much as a blind person dealing with the world, I can't fathom what it would be like. Closing my eyes is still not the same, despite that we spend half our lives with our eyes closed, whether through sleeping or blinking.

All in all, the original question can't be answered without unleashing a paradox. I may share certain aspects or traits with others, yet we never will be the same. As for the degree of 'severity' of Asperger's and anything beyond, the differences can be staggeringly diverse.

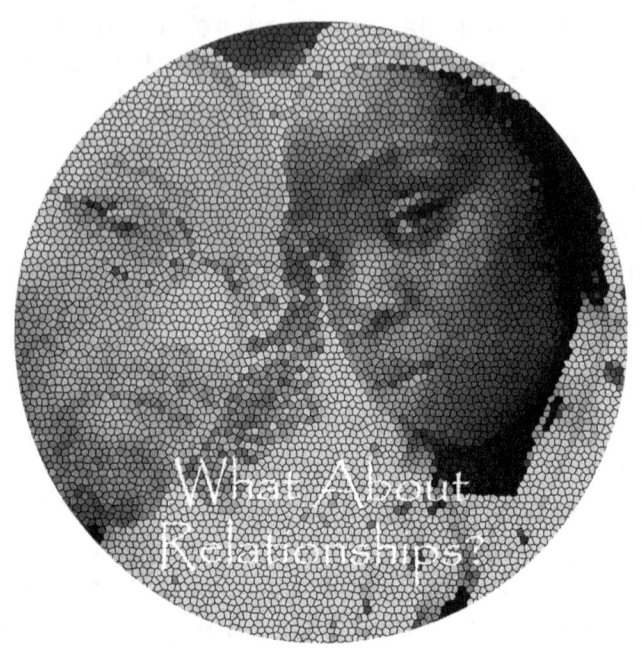

What About Relationships?

Appearing the same in most behaviours, you couldn't tell I am different from you. How could my wife have seen anything dissimilar when we met, or even after gotten married? What she knew about me, ironically, was through my writings I shared with her.

She never understood why I did certain things, or why they were as important to me as they were. Neither did I. I had never considered it could have been Asperger's, at least not seriously. I did at some point but dismissed the idea in favour of hyperactivity. That is another story altogether.

To be fair, my mother always overprotected me. I don't know if this was due to the fact that I was her youngest child or because she knew something. If that was the case, how do you tell your child he's not the same as others? One of the things she highly emphasized, at least with me, was that she would accept me the way I am. Although, that could have been because I didn't really date that much.

Dating is overrated. I always preferred solitude. I had some friends growing up (and have a few at this time), but spending time alone was never an issue for me. I never am bored, unlike most people who do get jaded.

Growing older was different from most, as I never made friends past high school. This excludes my current friends which I made in my late twenties in professional school, which I attended later on after University.

Afterwards, came my wife, who somehow was interested in getting to know more about me. Like most people, she didn't see anything special or unique in me, until she read love letters I wrote years prior to knowing her.

She was fascinated someone could orchestrate strings of words in such a way. I never thought much of it. It was what I was always used to, it was normal to me. It was never special, at least not to me. Others read them too and considered them to be deep, filled with sorrow and beauty. It's just what I do. I can't explain it, it comes easily.

Still, they weren't as beautiful as I wanted them to be, so I had to work on them, in which ended into a published work called 'Love Letter to Cleopatra'. For me, my writing is never good enough. While my wife could love something and find such soulful depth to it, it would still not be good enough. It can always be improved. I typically re-read everything at least four to five times before it is finalized.

Suffice it to say, I have charmed my wife with my craft, even though it was not destined to her. It perplexed me, as I've never loved someone because of their skills. Albeit, perhaps I am missing the mark; I suppose the soulful emotions behind the skill is what she considered.

On the other hand, for me, it's about how you make me feel. Just to be clear, I don't mean romantic feelings, but making me feel good as a person. I just want to feel special.

At the same time, this is hard to clarify as feelings can't be explained with so little words. For example, my wedding vows for my wife were around three pages double-spaced but could never contain an accurate depiction of any feelings I had for her. Yet, people loved those vows. For them, those were most definitely more than enough. Not me.

How can I explain to people that I could have done a better job, while improving upon the new foundation upon improving on the new foundation again? I realise it may not make much sense to people.

As for my wife, I gave her a chance to convince me she was worth my time. To be clear, it is much easier to allow potential friends to be part of your circle. If it doesn't work out, you can always go ahead and find a person or two to replace them. But your wife? It's not the same thing.

Your wife is the one who will be privy to a lot more. She will share the inner sanctum of a lot of things, and live through hell itself with you, just as much as you would with her. You can't just replace her as if it was that simple. Whether a life commitment, or a decade long affair, that person will share so much with you. The good, the bad and the ugly.

Whether you are planning on getting married, or in some instanced already married, that person seeks a lot from you in terms of what you can give them. Be it children with her, a house, a car, conversations and so on. The true test is knowing your own worth, while seeing what she sees in you. The question becomes: 'Why me?'

In truth, I have always been someone that lived in solitude, forsaking the idea of friendships for the most part. Most of my friends were always women, because typically men are just boring. I suppose the fact that I lived with my mom and sister may have had an impact on this as well. If I had to spend time with my wife and her sisters, I know a girls' night out would be better than spending time when a bunch of men who talk about cars, women and flight simulators.

When being single, the most common questions individuals wonder are: 'Why can't I find someone for me? Why can't I find that one person who would think more of me than just a friend or a good person?'

I too had wondered if I could find someone for me. My autobiography 'White, Canadian and Muslim' speaks more about this, in terms of why my wife was right for me. At the time, I wasn't seeking anyone, at least I had giving up on the idea at the time. Somehow, she found me.

As mentioned earlier, she saw nothing spectacular at first until she decided she wanted to know more about me. About what made me the person I am. She found a lot more than she bargained for. She discovered a well of emotions and feelings in the form of letters. As time went by, I flew down South to another country to propose to her.

We stayed in our respective places for around two years before getting married. During that time period, it allowed us to know more about each other. When she flew up North, I didn't want her to leave, even though I knew she had to go back before we could get married later.

Ironically, during the time when she was my fiancée, I was shocked to learn other women were interested in me, where they outright told me so. Some I had worked with in the past, and others I had known in prior scholarly Islamic events. That truly perplexed me.

It's not to say I am unlovable. For me, it was strange knowing that other women I had little interaction with at that point would suddenly tell me how they felt. That brought a degree of sadness in my heart, as I never wanted to be the cause of sadness in someone else because of how they felt about me.

At that point, I understood that there were desirable elements to me. My caring nature, my jovial personality, and my writing. Beyond that, there is something that is like a stonewall. Betrayal is not something I am good at. Typically, I am loyal, and in a relationship, that becomes a quality for the person you're with.

Marriage allowed me to understand a lot of things. For one, it enabled me to see family as more than just people in your life. I have always seen people as just people. Despite seeing television shows where family is everything, and they're there for each other, I never saw that in my family. I was wrong about that, as I understood that later in our marriage. I am still learning that.

As for her family, their interactions are tightly knit as they often communicate with each other. I have never been accustomed to that. I typically speak with my parents once a week, and my siblings, once in a while. When it comes to her family, I like to chime in. She calls it the peanut gallery when I do. I will surprise her one day with what that really means.

In terms of what marriage itself means, it brought me simple yet useful aspects to my life I otherwise lacked. For most, those may seem simplistic in what they represent. For me, marriage is about companionship more than anything. Do we do things like other couples? Sure, but for me the most important part of having someone in my life is the companion aspect of it.

We often engage in what you could call parallel play, whatever the equivalent is for adults. We'll do things on our own, while the other is nearby. Aside from that, we do the best we can to converse, watch some shows together, eat and so forth.

For her, doing activities is something she deems important. On the other hand, it isn't for me, although I will do what I can to make sure we do things. It would be unfair if she had to do everything by herself. I realise it isn't my forte, and so it's hard for me to plan out such activities.

If humankind spent millions of years creating an inside space to spend time in, clearly there must be a reason why this evolution took place. For our race to truly be different from animals that live in the wild, we created this inside space to protect ourselves from them and human predators. Down the line, we innovated through the ages, as we wanted to improve our lives and enjoyment of it. As the proverb goes: Necessity is the mother of invention.

Technology allows me to enjoy myself. It enables me to write, listen to music or even watch movies, and most importantly play videogames. That being said, the greatest lack for me was always companionship. It's true that there are certain benefits attached to such a company.

This is isn't to say that I wouldn't enjoy participating in the planned events her immediate family partakes in. Having access to her network and vice versa, has permitted us to learn more about ourselves.

Aside from the benefits of getting married, including the common ones I didn't list, there are obvious pitfalls. Nothing dramatic or sinister, simply things we wish were not frustrating but can be at times.

Usually, it's about silly arguments that break out. No yelling, screaming or name calling, simply admonishment. It can get tiring at times, but if not with her, then it would be with someone else. Whoever you're with, there will always be moments of tension.

I know this is something she doesn't understand, but I am incapable for the most part to be affirmative. It might be because I don't want to hurt her feelings, or since I can't speak her emotional language using the same vocabulary she uses. 'Yes' and 'no' are typically not part of my vocabulary when I deal with serious things. It may be more on the lines of 'I suppose', or 'I don't think so' or 'I don't know'.

It's neurologically hard for me to go ahead and use the words 'yes' and 'no'. It's like there's a part of my brain that cannot go ahead and use such words. It's a constant battle, and when she expects me to use either of those words, it creates a conflict within me.

It's hard to explain, as someone who wouldn't experience this couldn't really understand how difficult it would be to use certain words in clear-cut situations. It should obviously be simple, but because how my brain works, it becomes a taxing chore. Since I appear normal in most of my interactions, I think she expects me to always be capable of doing things that seem easy to her.

However, when I do say specific things in a precise manner, it repulses me and feels extremely awkward. It's not a feeling I enjoy experiencing. Bringing this into a real-world application, the closest example would be how people feel squeamish when they have to deal with spiders. The feeling itself isn't the same, but it's the closest one I can think of.

What makes things even harder for me, is when we get into an argument. It can feel so awkward. I understand her feelings get hurt, but what do you want me to do about it? I can't fix how she feels. Apologies are empty, or at least feel empty. As my sister used to tell me when we were in our late pre-teens and early teens: 'Excuse toi pas, fait attention!' (Don't apologize, just be careful!). That makes sense, as you wouldn't be in that situation if you were careful in the first place.

Apologies themselves are just a way of saying: 'Sorry if I don't know better; I'll try to do better next time. Chances are, I won't be different as to err is human, so I apologize in advance for being human'. Makes a whole lot of sense (sarcasm alert).

On the other hand, when she does something that I found annoying at the time, I'll be ok. Apologies mean nothing to me, as I placed that event behind me. I often forget what she's referring to when she apologizes later on. The apology in that situation is for her, not for me. I think it allows my wife to feel a sense of relief, in as much as she can move on past a negative experience.

If anything, the only apology and sense of urgency I would like for her to understand, would be when she accidentally hurts me physically. Physical pain is real. It has a real-world application which can be measured and quantified.

Mind you, all relationships are different, so other couples will experience things differently. One thing that I believe may be more common in these couples is how empathy is viewed. It's not that I don't care about her feelings or others' as human beings.

Rather, again, what do you want me to do about specific situations? For example, your dog died... ok? In that situation, a dog is not human. It's an animal. I will never understand that bond, ever. So I can't empathize with you. It's not because I hate or disrespect you, nor because you have less value to me than someone else. I just don't have the ability to understand, even if you try explaining it a thousand times. My response will always be: 'But... it's a dog. An animal'. In fact, it perplexes me when people refer to dogs as he/she. They're not human. You cannot humanize a non-human. Just as much as you cannot 'doganize' a non-dog (if that makes sense).

If another human being dies that I either didn't know or who didn't have a worldwide impact unlike Martin Luther King Jr. or Gandhi who did, then sure I can still feel bad for you. That being said though, I still won't feel a level of sadness. Again, it's not an ability I have. Since my brain cannot produce that emotion in circumstances that does not involve me. When my grandmother died, that was different, as she was the pillar of our family and I knew her personally.

The question a lot of people would have is: 'How can you not feel bad about XYZ situation? What's wrong with you?!' Nothing. The inability to perceive something means we cannot see the world the way you see it. Regardless of what happens, I can still acknowledge what you're saying and maybe reinforce it. To actually care about certain things is not something others like myself can do. Again, it's not about being good or bad. It's all about the neurological way our brain processes thoughts and feelings.

There is absolutely nothing anyone of us can do to modify that. It's not a behaviour. A behaviour would entail the ability to change after understanding XYZ. I can't change how my brain functions. Despite the ability to understand that something makes you feel a certain way, it doesn't mean I can understand the reasoning behind it.

For my wife, this can be frustrating at times. Since she is not like me, she has that capacity of understanding it's not my fault. Whenever I say or do something, she at times painstakingly comprehends this. I feel bad for her though, as I know it can be hard for her.

I am aware that 'treatments' exist. I find that offensive, as my personality and Asperger's is not something you can cure. I am who I am, and if someone has an issue with that, that's their problem, not mine. I have lived with myself with decades and I wouldn't change who I am because someone I don't know thinks I could be a 'better' version of myself.

Now, if you want cure anxiety or other potential side effects [for a lack of a better word] of Asperger's, that's different as anyone can suffer from such ailments.

All in all, living with someone with Asperger's can be a challenge. If you're someone without Asperger's reading this, and you're living with someone with Asperger's, refrain from criticizing them when you meet challenges head on.

Instead, use your ability to empathize and place yourself in his shoes. Imagine not having the same abilities as others. Skills you take for granted on a daily basis. Envision how he feels to live in a world where most people have a specific way of looking and acting in some situations. Imagine how hard it can be to be forced to accept that people expect you to do or say certain things. Something you take for granted, and which is far easier for you to deal with.

I can't pretend to be someone I'm not. Neither can the one in your life. All that said, he will possess far better qualities you would hope in a different partner. He'll most likely be loyal, sincere and genuine. If those aren't the best qualities in a relationship, I don't know what are, then.

Lastly, if you ever feel the need to cope with your partner, then think about how unfair that actually is. If you have the need to cope with who he is instead of accepting who he is, then you're doing it wrong. I live with my wife as we are married, so how fair would it be for either of us to cope with the other?

Coping means you have an issue living with someone with Asperger's. If anything, my wife and I have learnt to live with each other, through the best and the worst. We have legitimately gone through the worst situations life had to offer, all within a five-year span. We are together and doing the best we can to make sure we have an understanding and working through life together.

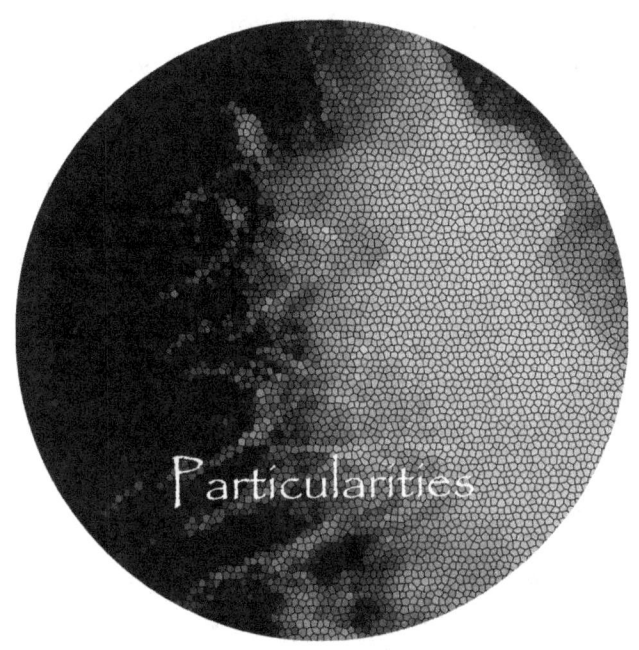

Particularities

Each person in the world is somehow unique. Nothing that sums us up is exactly the same as the next person or anyone else for that matter. Most people, however, have a certain number of things that coincide with how the majority of people do things. The easiest example is when you go to any restaurant, the knife is on the right side, and the fork on the left side.

That being said, I do things that people wouldn't understand. For the most part, I use logic to tell me how I should do things, I don't let societal norms dictate how I should do things. That would make zero sense, for good reason. Aside from this, my physical senses are different from others, as I am a lot more sensitive than the average person. On top of this, I need to do things a very specific way, while at other times, there are instances where I have a lot of trouble doing specific things.

Starting from the top, if we talk about food related matters, I eat with a spoon. I always have, and always will. This is something that I consider to be very natural.

While the majority of people would use a fork, I only use a fork with foods such as spaghetti. It baffles me when I see people using forks to eat foods that would be easier to grab with a spoon.

Spoons are made so you can place as much food in it without it falling through some of the holes, just as the ones found on forks. When I see people using a fork to eat macaroni and cheese for example, I will never understand how using a fork makes sense. Unless you're poking at it, as if using a pitchfork, what is the point of using one? A spoon is better suited for the purpose of grabbing as much macaroni and cheese as possible or any other foods for that matter.

I have never heard of any valid reason for using a fork aside from it being a preference. A preference for what though? Not eating as efficiently as possible? That's how I see. A tad arrogant, to be sure. Being the only person eating with a spoon at a table, I feel bad for the ones around me not knowing the joys of using a spoon.

As for placing the fork on the left side and knife on the right side, why? Etiquette? Etiquette of what?

Complicating your life? Let's be honest here, there is no valid reason for this at all. As mentioned earlier, I use logic to tell me how to operate. This is not logical, unless you're left-handed of course.

Most people are right-handed, and so they eat using their fork/spoon with their right hand. Why is the fork/spoon on the left side, then? I know of no one who can give me a valid reason. Dinning etiquette is not a reason, and certainly less a valid one.

What I am saying and how it comes off as may seem arrogant, but it's not. Here's why: Most of my life people always asked why I eat with a spoon, as well as trying to correct me when I would place the knives on the left side. What is arrogant, is for others to assume that they know better than me.

They don't. I use logic, and logic dictates how I operate make sense. Having people constantly tell me I am wrong about something I know for a fact I am right about is beyond frustrating. For me, there is no greater pet peeve than being told I am doing it wrong when it comes to utensils. Next time you are at a restaurant, take the fork in your left hand. After all, if the fork is on the left side, shouldn't you use your left hand? Afterwards, tell me if it feels natural.

As you can tell, I am very touchy about this subject, and it's because most of my life people have sought to correct what they saw as an incorrect behaviour. I disliked them for that and hated their behaviour. How I eat is not a behaviour, it's the logical way to eat. Why should I let some erroneous dinning etiquette dictate how I eat? No, I will never kowtow to such a behaviour.

I don't need people to tell me how to perform any basic human task, as I find offense in people assuming I can't live my life correctly. I know how to eat, shower and sleep, thank you very much!

There is one particularity that my wife doesn't understand but has learnt to accept. It's something that used to irritate her to no end. I will mix my food together. Mashed potatoes and steak? No problem! Cut up the steak, mix it with the mashed potatoes and use a spoon to savour the goodness of those two flavours together!

I do that for everything. I can't explain why. It just tastes better like that. It doesn't make much sense for me to separate the food I'm eating. Sure, each has its particular flavour, yet they acquire a better, unique taste once you mix them. I know most people don't do this, but you should give it a try. Except broccoli. I eat those as are, since... it's broccoli. Not the greatest taste, and its shape is odd.

Another particularity includes my sensitivity. My skin itches all the time because I am ultrasensitive. I have read in multiple sources that people with Asperger's tend be hypersensitive. It's annoying to no end. Imagine wearing something slightly too small. You wouldn't think much of it, but for me, my body would feel like it's being tickled.

Unless I am laser focused doing something, I tend to scratch myself often. Living like that is extremely difficult. Whether you're talking about clothing detergent, dry air, slightly smaller clothes or anything else, those have an impact on me.

Aside from my skin giving me endless grief, sound is another sense that is extremely heightened. I have learnt to drown most of it out though. There are others that always startle me, and I cringe every moment I hear those sounds.

When my wife drops something on the floor, I just tense up and shriek. Most people wouldn't even hear much, except the actual clang of the object hitting the floor. I hear the clang, but I also feel the reverberation of the noise that is made. It feels so loud and it hurts my ears.

I can hear things that the majority of people can't hear. Although, voices are different, as those need to be clearer for me to understand. Still, there are instances where I'm able to know if there is no noise around. I do recall one instance when I was a child in class. My classmate was maybe five metres away from me, and she whispered to the teacher that she had to go to the bathroom. I heard that, even though she was whispering, and five metres away.

Since my hearing is more sensitive than the majority, it has become both a nuisance and an advantage. When my mother and I lived together before I moved out, we lived on the top floor of a house. When she'd go out, I knew every time she was home. Through two walls and her car doors, I heard when she geared in the emergency break.

Every. Single. Time. Without fault. I would go to the window to see if it was her or someone in another car.

From my current uppermost apartment floor level, I can even hear the elevator's voice when it says it's on the parking level. I can't explain why I have such sensitive hearing, but it's odd that I can hear things no one else can. Having heightened senses is one of those things that can be both good and bad. For all intent and purposes, I have learnt to drown out most of it.

As if this wasn't enough, I suffer from what's called the photic sneeze reflex. Whenever I go outside and the sun is shining, I am almost guaranteed to sneeze. In fact, I have sneezed every single day of my life as far as I can remember. It's annoying.

Since the velocity of a sneeze is more than a hundred and fifty kilometres according to the American Lung Association, it physically tires me out. That is way faster than a speeding car. I could be wrong, but I believe some of my sneezes may be faster, as I know of no one else who gets tired after sneezing. When this happens, it feels like my body has emptied itself of every single air molecule inside. There has been so many times where my sneezing has severely scared others.

My favourite example of this was when I was in the car with my mother. I sneezed, and the pedestrian crossing the street jumped and screamed. That sometimes happens. Other times people look at me, wondering what the hell that was.

Another thing which I can notice is the taste between organic milk and non-organic milk. Trust me, the average person can't tell the difference. I can, and organic milk is definitely better taste wise. I could probably tell the difference between other foods if I looked for it, but don't really care to.

Being hypersensitive is one of those things that you can't explain. It just is. Most of the time, it can be frustrating and annoying, because it becomes a nuisance. Other times, it can be good or at the very least give me a cue that something is either happening or will happen.

For example, I know when I am getting a cold. I can feel my body tell me I will be sick. It doesn't literally speak to me of course, although it does act a certain way which enables me to know that it's either coming, or that I can try preventing it from occurring. The latter doesn't work that often. I can read my body's cues in such a situation, even though they appear so minimal at best. The average person could not read those cues, as they're not even classified as symptoms per se.

All of this aside, I have other particularities that have more to do with who I am and how my brain works. There are specifically three things that I can't help doing or desiring for to happen. I am sure there are others, but these three are the worthiest.

Usually when someone tells you you're good at something, the typical response is to say thank you. Not mine. The below explains my thought process, in a raw form. It won't be polished; it rather will explain how I view such a situation. A trigger for me is when someone tries to correct what they perceive as erroneous behaviour. Again, the below will show my frustration with this as I explain the why.

If another is merely acknowledging I am good at something, why should I thank them for noticing my talent? When somebody tells me I am good at something, my response is simply: 'I know'. There is nothing malicious in this, although it does perplex a lot of people. It's exasperating when someone tries to correct me by saying I should say thank you. No. I won't. When I pray to Allah, I thank Him for my gift. I will never thank another human for my talent.

On the other hand, if you want to tell me what I wrote is nice, well written and so on, I will say thank you for that. That by itself is a compliment. There is a difference by complimenting my writing and saying positive things about it, versus telling me I am a good writer or computer tech.

I understand people don't see a difference in either situation. I do. I'm fully aware that others will never fathom this. For me, it is a world of a difference. In truth, it perplexes me when other individuals believe they should be thanked when acknowledging a gift that they have not given. This is the equivalent of you thanking your neighbour for the gift your husband gave you. This obviously makes zero sense, and that's the same way I feel.

As mentioned earlier, I operate through logic. If something makes no sense, I won't abide by such a societal etiquette. Neurotypical individuals may outnumber non-neurotypicals, but it doesn't mean those individuals are correct. At times, my responses are so atypical for the neurotypical, that they don't always know how to respond afterwards.

My advice for you is the following: Let go of your perceptions. Let go of what you know is right. Imagine this, when a car speeds to a certain extent, the wheels appear like they are going the other way. You brain, in that situation, believes that the wheels could only be is that position if it's going backwards. And so, it forces your eyes to see, ironically, the wrong truth.

Let go of what society expects of you or me. Once you can see that there are other truths to a situation, it will allow you to understand that people can have ideas that are either just as good or even better. As you let go, you will be capable of letting go of that mould.

When I walk in my neighbourhood, all I see are houses that look the same, because they have the same mould. Just like architecture, we are meant to be different. Once you break free from it, you'll experience a world that you can shape to the person you are. Don't let the world mould you, instead be the one to shape it.

The instant you're capable of seeing beyond it, will be the moment which enables you to perceive a way of thinking that was always there but never considered. There is no one better placed than someone with Asperger's to understand this, as we constantly have to deal with people who all have a different worldview than ours.

If you are willing to enter that world and see how freeing it can be, I encourage you to eat with a spoon, to even try real hard to see the taste difference between milk and organic milk, or even close your eyes and hear the sounds around you. All of that to say, enter the world of someone different, and walk a kilometre in his shoes.

We have to do it every day, to a certain extent. Now it's your turn to be us and see what we see and perceive what we notice. Force yourself to feel what we feel, so you may be kinder and more understanding to someone like us. You may then consider that your normal isn't so normal after all. You may finally see that my normal is simply normal.

There are, however, other aspects of me which many would have a hard time understanding. I tried explaining the next point to my wife, yet I don't think she'll ever understand. With a French speaker, I need to speak French with them, and the same is true with an English speaker.

What? That's probably the word you just used. It makes no sense, and it doesn't to me either. Yet, I feel an extreme sense of repulsion when I force myself to speak French to a non-French speaker – the same goes for English. I can't explain it, this is just the way my brain is wired. Although, I can speak either to someone whose mother tongue is neither.

There is a part of how my brain is wired that tells me to speak the correct language. I don't know why my brain functions the way it does. This is definitely one of those things I wish I didn't have to endure, as this has become problematic at times with my wife. It makes it harder for me to help her learn French, among other things.

Attempting to help her, I feel a sense of repulsion to use French words with her. It feels like selective mutism, but with a language instead. It's definitely aggravating, as I would love to not feel the way I do. Unfortunately, there's nothing I can do about it.

Perhaps one day she will understand that sense of cringe that creeps up my spine. The same is true with my family. I will be on the phone with my sister for example, and she'll speak English, but I'll respond in French. The fact she'll speak English doesn't bother me, but I need to respond in French when speaking with her.

How can you explain this to someone who doesn't experience such a strange feeling, which even to me, makes no sense? I thought this was something I just experienced with my family, until I met my wife. I then realised that this wasn't the case. Before I understood I had Asperger's, I believed this would be something that would go away.

Since I have Asperger's, this is something that will stay with me. There is nothing I can do to change this. After all, I am the person I am. Perhaps one day, with age, this will change as well. I mean, everyone changes to a certain extent. Who knows, maybe this will also be one of those. For the moment, however, I will have to deal with this the best I can. Hopefully in time, my wife will continue learning French with her sister.

In any event, there is a third trait which is very particular to say the least. You have to be to my left. You want to cuddle with me? You have to be on my left. You want to walk beside me? You need to walk to my left. You're in the same bed as me? You need to sleep to my left.

It's not even a personal preference, it's just that my brain forces me to prefer that a person is to my left. I can do any of those on my right, but there's such an awkwardness to it, that is feels forced and unnatural.

I have my own spot on my couch which in this case, ironically, is on the left side, as it was chosen because of the fact of my surroundings. On some rare occasions, I'll sit on the right side if I need to do something very specific. For all intent and purposes, I'll sit on the left side, and if my wife and I cuddle during a movie, it feels so unnatural to use the right side of my body, including my arm around her.

I've never given it much thought as to why this was ever important to me. I thought it could have been a defence mechanism of some sort. This by itself does make sense, since I am right-handed. But knowing what I now know, this is probably not the case. It's just that my brain is wired in this way.

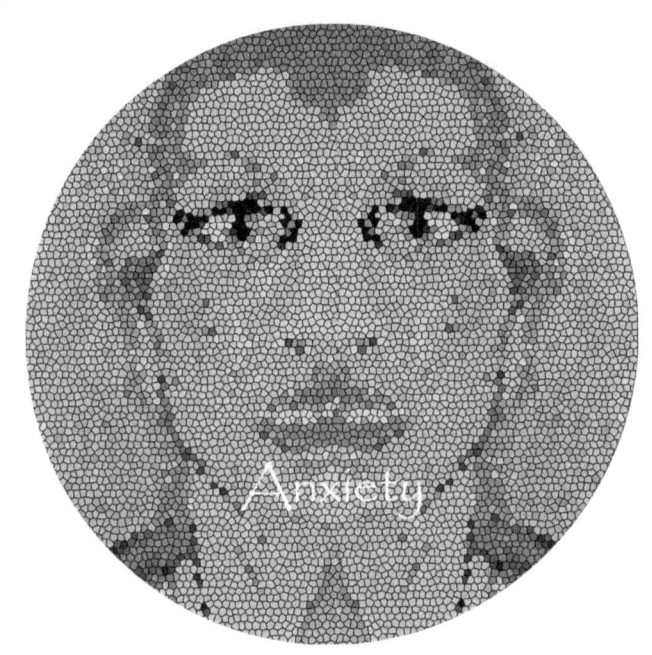

It's safe to assume that everyone knows what anxiety is, and how crippling it can be. Imagine feeling that way every single day. Through the worst and the bad, that dreaded sensation surges. The body expresses something so dire, that even sleep itself doesn't remove that ailment, as you wake up from a half-sleep. I pray to Allah to remove such a state from my mind, but I still don't know how that will come, nor when.

As far as I am aware, people with Asperger's tend to have increased anxiety compared to neurotypical individuals. What is the reason for that? It might simply be because of how the brain is wired. All we have at this point when it comes to Asperger's are hypotheses. Otherwise, we could easily get rid of some of the most undesirable traits like anxiety.

I don't know how a neurotypical person feels anxiety and the degree that he perceives it. The way I do is a most gnawing sensation. I feel like a can't breathe very well, while feeling this sensation in my stomach, as if it's trying to process something. Visualize this every single day of your life, how terrible this would be.

Normally, for anxiety, exercise helps. In my case, despite exercising most days for around half an hour, it doesn't help much. Ironically, that is the best way as far as I know in terms of dealing with anxiety. Another way to deal with this affliction would be to meditate or stay in a state of deep calmness.

I can't. I am incapable of sitting still for very long. Despite sitting down as I'm writing, I'm still moving something consistently (my arms and fingers), or even my legs. Telling me to meditate makes absolutely no sense. It should, right? But, I have never been able to sit still. This will be explained later, as the reason will make sense.

My brain is constantly thinking about something, and at some point, one of those things is bound to make me anxious. Anxiety is like a constant companion, a constant fear. A constant. It's like your best friend turned rogue on you. As if vilified in a single moment. If anything, I tend to do different things, like writing, playing videogames, watching movies, or exercising.

Whatever I can do to keep that fiend at bay, I do the best that I can do. It's not always easy to deal with the world around, while dealing with your own fears. It's the equivalent of living two lives at once. A past, present and future that comes together to bring you down, while still having to consider another world around you that won't understand how you are.

That is a burden not easily dealt with, or forgotten for that matter. Yet, I am learning to better myself which, one day hopefully, will allow me to rely on no one but myself. What anxiety does is tell you that you can't do XYZ because of the fear from within.

It's a wolf that comes at you, trying to make you believe that you can't accomplish some of your goals. Albeit, some of those are because of Asperger's which creates a barrier preventing you from doing certain things. As for the actual fears brought out by anxiety, it creates a wall of fear, without a way out.

Without a door to exit through, you're faced with either cowering in the corner like so many have done, or to conquer them one at a time. If that is even possible? Give them a cookie, it might occupy those wolves?

Regardless of this, the best way to deal with these is when your partner supports you. You won't always see eye to eye, nor agree on how to do things. The most important thing is to listen. I listen to my wife, even though she doesn't always think I do. Listening doesn't mean I'll do something right now.

If anything, it means I'll consider what she has to say.

Some of her advice are good, while others not as much. Since I have Asperger's, I don't always see the world the way she does. Hence why I don't always see her advice as good. When it's tailored for a world that sees itself a certain way, I can't be expected to share that same way of thinking.

Instead, I can feel overwhelmed. That sensation is nothing short of your mind shutting down from processing information, and rejecting it altogether. It can transform itself into what is called sensory overload. Basically, it's the feeling of being overwhelmed by your surroundings or inputs like noise for example.

Sensory overload can become the number one fear where advice will never change anything. For all intent and purposes, crowds are synonymous with sensory overload. A person with Asperger's like myself needs time by himself. Be it to recharge myself or being far from obnoxiously loud individuals who only seem to make it their life's work to be as loud as possible. What may seem like a lot of time to spend in solitude, isn't enough for me.

I could spend days on end by myself and still not have enough time for myself. To the neurotypical individual, that makes no sense. That's ok, but it does make a lot of sense to me and countless others with Asperger's.

Even though I am married, my wife and I spend considerable time on our own, working on our crafts. For my wife, I believe it has to do with me achieving my higher end goals. As long as I work at it, she seems more thrilled by that than time spent with her on a more mundane activity. But when we spend time together, at least we are freer to spend more lavishly on a specific activity, whatever that may be.

Due to my inability of spending time in large crowds, it prevents me from doing a lot of things. Which, ironically, I mostly couldn't care less about anyhow. So, not much of a loss there. Still, there are events or places my wife would like to attend or go to. As for me personally, home sweet home. I could spend most of my life indoors, and I'd have no issues with that.

However, the biggest event that brings real fear in my heart is one surrounded by a lot of people as you know. When my wife and I go to the mosque during special events, I feel a high degree of anxiety. I wish this wasn't the case, as I know how much those events mean to my wife. It means less to me, since my primal concern relates to the absence of anxiety.

Even when I went to the church in the early two thousand ten's with mom to commemorate my grandfather's death in the nineties, I felt so uncomfortable. Mind you, there wasn't a lot of people in there, as normally churches in Quebec are fairly empty anyhow.

In this instance, there might have been a few reasons, such as the fact that there were people, and because I am not Christian and thus felt out of place. Still, there was a level of anxiety and intense awkwardness when I saw everyone go for the representation of the body of Christ. Being the only one behind, and thus a certain amount of attention placed on me, felt very awkward.

Of course, there are other instances that affect me in different ways. For example, I loathe going to the dentist, as I anticipate the potential pain. I don't mind talking one-on-one with the hygienist. They're always sweet. The point though, is that the fear of something is real. It's never about bravery, cowardice or anything else.

Truly, there is no way of explaining what fear feels like. I may be slightly squeamish with some spiders, but I'll never understand the deathly scared expressions and reactions of others who are absolutely frightened by spiders. Ultimately, fright cannot be explained. You can't imagine how I feel about certain things, nor can I know how you feel. At best, we can make an educated assumption, nothing more.

That being said, we are who we are. As far as I know, anxiety is not something you can cure with bravery. I wish this was a roleplaying game, where we could take different types of potions for a variety of debilitating ailments. Low on health? Take a health potion! Low on bravery? Take a remove fear potion! It would be nice, but life doesn't work that way.

True, there are always a thousand and one medications you can take. Here in Canada, we have both Canadian and American television channels. Whenever they advertise medications in the United States, it always goes something like this: 'Suffering from anemia? Take Anemia-No-More! Side effects include stomach cramps, partial hearing loss, heightened skin sensitivity causing itching, may cause swelling in your legs and possible bladder shyness. May also increase the possibility of getting tuberculosis'. What? Get rid of one ailment to get another twenty? Wait, what? Tuberculosis?! No.

I certainly don't want to be one of those people who take medication just because. My mother takes medication for XYZ, and I feel bad for her. The same goes for anyone else taking multiple medications. Maybe those people prefer taking all that medication. I don't know.

That being said, what is considered Western medicine is very destructive. Our system focuses on destroying the cause instead of healing the body. If you weren't aware of that, let that sink in. the best example is chemotherapy. With all the technology we have, you'd think we'd have a better alternative than killing bad and good cells. Let's make the body weaker first, before healing it.

If anything, I do remember taking a few items through the science of naturopathy. That helped me when it came to anxiety, although I forgot what they were called. I do know that natural remedies are best suited when it comes to anxiety. Sometimes, that's still not enough.

Part of removing anxiety is to take some natural remedies, while exercising, and calming your body. Despite doing all this, it's not always sufficient and is extremely time consuming. Unlike a normal form of anxiety, the one I suffer from feels more debilitating as it's coupled with the knowledge that the world can't accept me for how I am. What people don't understand, they either fear or mock.

All in all, living within a neurotypical world is the equivalent of living in a harsh climate. With nothing but a desolate land to grow crops. You do the best that you can, yet your best is never enough. If it was, we would all be as highly successful as my favourite Tech Expert, Bill Gates, with the same drive, ingenuity and brilliance that he showed when he shaped a part of our future.

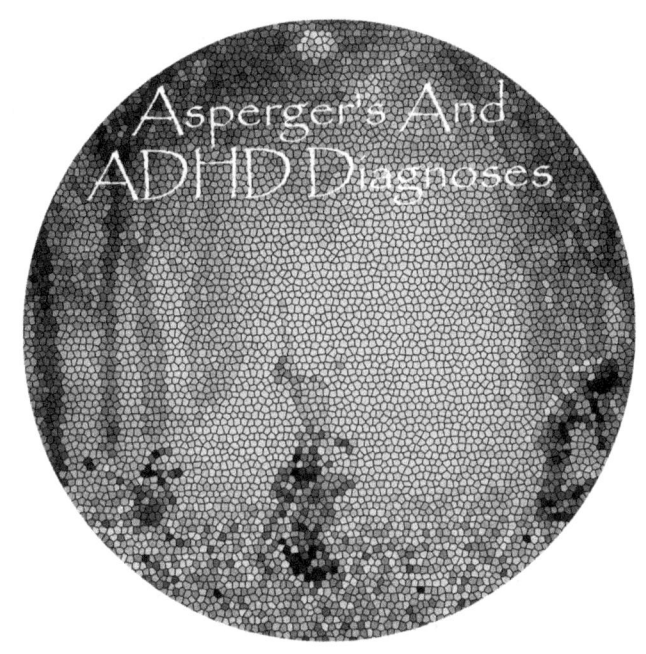

Asperger's And ADHD Diagnoses

Are you from my generation? If so, you may have Asperger's. Of course, I don't know how old you are, nor what generation you're from. What I can speak about is mine. My generation is the one that saw the revival of the videogame industry. The one that saw the rise of the personal computer with ridiculously low specs compared to what we use now. We saw the rise of operating systems. And an increase in the use of glasses.

On the negative side of this, however, we saw accidental recklessness in doctors. Not because they were bad, nor because they didn't know what they were doing. Instead, we saw the rise of methylphenidate prescriptions handed out like candy (methylphenidate is not a brand name. Use a search engine to find more about the brands associated with this). The fault was not the manufacturers', as their medications had an intended purpose, which they fulfilled.

The fault lies with the doctors who either did not have the correct training, or who were unaware of the difference between Attention Deficit Hyperactivity Disorder and Asperger's Syndrome. To a certain degree, both have similar symptoms for a lack of a better word.

Perhaps the fault lied with the parents who did not know better, or the doctors for not referring the parents to a specialist, so they may diagnose the child with a more appropriate diagnosis. Regardless, this definitely screwed up a lot of peoples' lives.

Imagine not knowing why you are the way you are, while having a lesser ability to deal with people. Visualize either being married and then divorced, or having your best friend having stopped talking to you among a myriad of other potential scenarios. All of this could have been avoided if you just knew. Unless you study psychology and psychiatry, there is no reason for you to delve into the medical field, as there is so much to learn. You'd overwhelm yourself, and in the process develop hypochondriasis.

Suffice it to say that knowing something can make you understand, and especially your partner, why you do things the way you do things. That day you emotionally hurt them, it wasn't because you wanted to hurt their feelings. It was either because you didn't realise at all that you would, or because you were oblivious to that fact.

This has definitely happened with my wife, but she's gotten better at understanding that whenever I do or don't do something, it's not because I don't care about her feelings. I'm just oblivious to the fact that XYZ matters to her, even if she tells me a thousand times. All of this to say that a wrong diagnosis by a medical professional is life changing and eye opening for your partner.

Consider that for a moment: For the last three decades of your life, you could have understood why you do some of the things you do; you could have not been on medication while a child, which is a hard thing to forgive as that changed your entire childhood; you could have had better support tailored for Asperger's instead of something you probably don't even have – ADHD.

A part of me wants to blame my mother, as she didn't know what to do. Another part of me feels bad for her, as her brother Jean-Pierre had autism (though I don't know how bad), and her nephew René (my cousin) has severe autism – he looks and sounds like a mere child, despite being older than me.

Maybe she was trying to get as far from that type of diagnosis as possible. I get it, this would be a situation you pray never comes. Where your son remains a child forever, trapped inside an ever-growing body, with a five-year-old mind.

If anything, my love for the past contains my memories in a bubble from twenty years ago, which for everyone else was way back in the nineties. For me, those were like yesterday. Most of the movies and music I listen to are from the eighties and nineties. But my actual mind has grown, as it will continue to do so.

Aside from this tendency to hold onto art from a bygone era, my Asperger's – in neurotypical terms – is so mild, that I appear like anyone else. I don't know of anyone who would even know that I have Asperger's unless they're professionals and know what to look for.

For all intent and purposes, I am neurotypical for most people (except, again, professionals who know what to look for). I think she was afraid, since only boys were affected on her side of the family. I do believe that Asperger's Syndrome and Autism are only passed from the opposite gender. So, a mother to her son for example. This would confirm it in this case.

Unfortunately, teachers and doctors back then were quick to label children as hyperactive. Children are meant to have energy. That is not hyperactivity, it's called being a child. Having energy is not a sickness. I don't respect parents who believe that their children should take medication because they believe their children have hyperactivity.

This erroneous and uninformed thinking is what ruined part of my childhood. I think that for my mother, it was an exit she could take, being relieved of something far sinister than she feared. If your child is having issues at school, consider the fact that the school does not correctly tailor their approach to multiple types of children.

In fact, consider that the problem may not be related to your child, but to the teacher's view of how a child should behave. Again, children are meant to have energy. I personally don't believe hyperactivity exists in children. In adults, yes, as I've seen it. As for children, they have energy and are meant to expend that energy through activities. That is simple nature at work.

Doctors are not miracle workers. Always get a second opinion from a trained psychologist or psychiatrist who specializes in things like Asperger's Syndrome to rule out the possibility of that being the case. I understand that parents don't always know what to do, and they seek out help. That's fine, in fact that's the responsible thing to do.

As I was on medication when I was younger, my way of being felt like I was a zombie. Anyone in my grade could attest to this. Those types of medications change how you are. It's frightening. I hated the way I was. At some point in high school, I told my mom I was not going to take the medication anymore. I became normal again.

The diagnosis of ADHD feels like a death sentence. The change of behaviour and personality is disgusting under those medications. It radically alters the person you are, robbing you of your way of being and your personality.

If I was able to graduate from University in an extremely difficult subject matter, I did something right. Medications like the above don't fix who you are, nor improve you. They zombify you, making teachers see you as either less disruptive or less of a wandering mind among other things. Did I need these to graduate from High School, CEGEP or University? Nope.

No one had the right to tell me I wasn't good enough. Ultimately, telling your child they need to take medication to be a certain way is an acknowledgment that something is wrong with them, and they're not good enough to accomplish academic goals on their own. But there isn't anything wrong with them. They most likely have Asperger's, and what they need is a tailored teacher for them who understands Asperger's and knows how to act with a child with Asperger's.

Even today as an adult, looking at Asperger's, my mind wanders off. When my wife talks to me, I sometimes think about something else and have no clue what she said. It certainly isn't because I wasn't paying attention. I was, but somewhere down the line, my mind wandered off and started thinking about something else. This isn't ADHD. It's Asperger's. I do have trouble paying attention to her at times, and again, this is Asperger's.

I can't help it, it's part of who I am. I don't tell her my mind wandered off, as I know it would hurt her feelings, despite the fact that I can't help it. Words themselves are meaningless, as they are mere shapes and sounds when spoken. They are, however, powerful nonetheless as we attach meanings to them, somehow.

The person I am is not fixable, as there is nothing wrong with me, yet due to the nature of who I am, it has an impact on the person I'm with. Finally knowing I had Asperger's made my wife understand me quite a deal more.

On top of this, I have a certain degree of energy that most likely exasperates others around me. This may explain why children want me to do activities with them. I'm like a big kid, who enjoys fun activities. Although typically for me, that includes videogames, but sports like soccer or badminton are fun too. I guess tag is ok too. You can't catch me!

Normally for me, this level of energy manifests itself in a way where I seek attention from my wife. It becomes fairly difficult to remain quiet when she's doing something important or even when she's talking to her family. In those instances when using her laptop, it's better if she's working in the bedroom or on the dinning room table. That is, when I myself am gaming in the living room. Otherwise, I will constantly talk to her. It's one of those 'I can't help it' moments.

It's very difficult for me to keep quiet. Mind you, I rarely talk. But when I do, boy do I ever! About random things that make no sense! I just talk to say things, like a random keynote speaker no ones wants to hear in the peanut gallery. When we do have a serious conversation, well that's another ball game. I always have something insightful to say.

Something else to consider with me when it comes to attention, I always need to be doing something. It's impossible for me to just sit still without something to do. If I'm writing, I need to listen to music. If doing literally any other task or activity, I need to have something in the background. Be it music or a television show. Typically, Stargate™ or Star Trek™ which normally plays on television.

The necessity to consistently have that need, means I will never just sit idly by. I could, although I would constantly be trying to find something else to do. While others may need to always be surrounded by others, I just need my activities and I'll be fine. As strange as it may seem, that would even include opening the fridge door. Of all things I could be doing, let me look for food I won't even eat. You know at that point I really have nothing better to do.

All of that to say that I have a lot of energy, while also having a mind that constantly has wheels spinning at an infinite rate. That includes whenever I sleep as well. The wheels keep on turning. I am incapable of not having a thought, thinking about anything, or even something completely random. To fill any empty gaps, I'll even create small ballads, songs and so forth just to keep my mind occupied. Mind you, my brain never seems to want to sleep. My body yes, but my brain would like nothing further than that.

This is both a blessing and a curse. It allows me to be very creative and inventive, without allowing me to have a moment of peace and quiet without a care in the world. In the end, my mind wanders off as it always tries to create new experiences for me. For example, when I was younger, I had created a fantasy world but never had the chance to edit that work. The creativity within that series is immense, and the potential is limitless. There is a reason for how my brain is wired. It allows me to tap into a well of promising and raw human power.

For others who would have me think that I ever had ADHD, and who sought to silence my energy and voice, did not know or understand what power the human brain is capable of. The creativity, inventiveness and unlimited thought process are things which can be unleashed to no end. Allah created us in a specific way for a reason. All of us have the potential to release an untapped source of influence from within. To silence that power is dangerously reckless.

I was the way I was and still am for a valid reason. It allows me to be different, while possessing the talents I do. The same can be said of others. We need to nurture our gifts, and drown out those who would seek to discourage us. What society doesn't understand, it burns it at the stake (figuratively at this point). Society is frightened of what it cannot understand.

All we can do is embrace our uniqueness instead of the monotonous drones we could be. That will enable us to force the world to accept us. As time goes on, we as societies, have learnt to grow more accepting. We still have a long way to go, at least we are not literally burning people at the stake anymore.

At the end of the road, despite sharing some traits with ADHD, Asperger's is undeniably different. It shapes the person you are. It moulds the normalcy that outlines the individual you are. It's not a sickness, nor something to regulate. I am the person I am with both strengths and weaknesses, as well as the occasional oddity here and there.

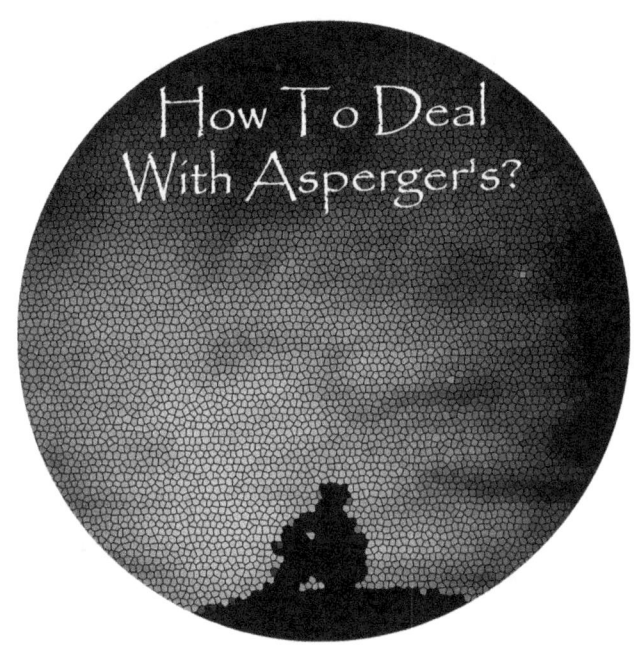

How To Deal With Asperger's?

Before answering that specific question, we need to determine if Asperger's is an issue. To the neurotypical individual, they seek to always fix things they deem broken, or outright throw them away. Asperger's doesn't diminish my intellectual or motor capacities at all. If anything, it shapes the person I am, as well as shapes the way I see the world around me through mainly two lenses: Logic vs the illogic.

It enables me to perceive what the world should really be like. One where we are all equal, regardless of gender, colour, language or religion. The rest of the world, as I've seen, seem to think otherwise. Due to my nature, I have a more neutral world view.

Even though many may see me as atypical, my nature of seeing logic on a greener earth makes me more typical than atypical. If anything, the way I perceive my surroundings better equips me to see myself as normal. As I see the world around me as abnormal, I often am perplexed concerning a lot of the hate that exists.

Due to this, I don't identify as an outlier. Therefore, there is nothing wrong with me, and nothing to fix. Dealing with Asperger's would mean there is something wrong with me. There is nothing for me to correct. The reality is that since I think and do things differently, it only means I am different from a lot of people.

To assume there is something wrong with difference is where intolerance comes into play. The sad truth is the fact that a lot of people use gender, colour, language and/or religion to push discriminatory agendas. Difference is what makes the world go round.

After all, mathematics and coffee (potentially) are Arabic, numbers Roman, hockey Canadian and so on and so forth. Without the diverse nations on earth, the human race may not be as advanced as it is at this point. All this to say that perceiving someone like me as different, special or whatever adjective you want to employ, makes that person discriminatory towards me.

Without knowing how someone sees the outside world, or how his thought process is, how can someone else make a judgement of that individual?

Any of us may look down at someone else with down syndrome or a person who is extremely low functioning autistic and think to ourselves: 'Man, is that person ever miserable. How can they even be happy?' For all we know, ignorance of the complexities of this world is truly bliss. If anything, Allah gave them a glimpse of Jannah (Heaven), where they know of no such dreadful complexity in the world.

That's what makes you think about how the world revolves around its own ignorance. Where our knowledge of our surrounding is like a grain of sand on this earth. We are nothing but one of the lowest, common, finite denominators in this ever-expanding universe. We are nothing compared to the vastness of this universe, but our egos are just as big. Due to this, we believe we have the right to be superior, when in fact we are nothing.

That being said, there's nothing to be done with Asperger's, as it allows me a more neutral way of seeing things and seeing the world for what it is. Sometimes, this is something others fail to comprehend. Like when my wife apologizes for something she perceived as wrong. It still won't change the situation that happened. The way I may have felt for an instant, is merely a fleeting moment in the billions of years that the universe has existed. It is not worth the trouble for me to worry about.

To be sure, I not only have a specific way of seeing things, I also have a way of doing things. In religions in general, we regard what people do on a daily basis as rituals. The easiest example would be the act of praying or Wudu (ablutions – cleaning yourself before praying). Those are considered rituals, as you do those everyday, while the act itself being repetitious. The same, however, can be said of a hockey or basketball player who does something very specific before playing a game.

Others would call those routines, but from the perspective from someone like myself who Majored in Islam (technically Eastern Religions), I can guarantee you that it's not a routine. A routine is when you have breakfast at eight in the morning, every morning. When it's something that you do because you must do it for X reason, that's a ritual. Not starving yourself is not a ritual.

There are a variety of things I do because I have to do them. Excluding ablutions and praying, I get up in the morning, play half an hour of an MMO (Massively Multiplayer Online game), then I start writing. Those are types of rituals that can change if the need is required or if desired. Otherwise, I always check in with my fleet-mates in the MMO I play with, through a social app. Whether I post something or not is a different matter.

Adding all of this together and the person I am, doesn't really say much about who I am or what I do. During the course of a day, I have a pretty simple life. I get up, eat (most days), play an MMO, check with them, and write. Later, I either game a bit or do something random. Afterwards, I eat supper, exercise, and go work overnight.

Even though I can't speak for others with Asperger's, I don't need a lot to occupy myself. Simply put, all my energy I have is placed into the creative arts. I write, I sing (terribly, mind you), and I recently started composing/mixing music because I would eventually like to expand my love of creativity in every imaginable possible way. Creating videos is next on my list.

I love art that is provocative, dark and mesmerising. As well as funny and smart. To me, those convey a sense of reality, since those are the best way to communicate with others. Art tells others how we think, as well as how we perceive the best way to convey our feelings to them. If anything, this is how I deal with myself.

As for Asperger's itself, it's not a disease, an accident or anything else for that matter. It's part of who I am, not what I am. The reality for others and myself is how we deal with each other. That is the real question.

I've never had that many friends. Only four at a time, even now. Always has been four. Different ones in different periods of my life, mind you. Still, only four. In all of this, I don't believe I ever treated any of my friends poorly, yet I do believe that a lot of people get offended by me or just don't like certain aspects of me. How we deal with each other is what charms or angers individuals.

Frankly, I don't care at all if some people don't like me or what I do or say. I don't live my life for them. Besides, because I have Asperger's, my approach to others may be perceived as a bit abrasive at times. I know I have hurt people's feelings, but it was never out of malice or anything as such. Often in such a situation, people react in anger, name-calling and the likes. I've learnt to ignore people in such situations, as it is pointless to reply to juvenile behaviour.

They act in a very childish manner. They can't handle the fact that someone like myself does not respond to the world around them the same way they think I should, and resort to juvenile behaviour instead of trying to understand. There's always a reason for what someone says, but not attempting to understand their side is childish. Mind you, some people are just jerks, and reasoning with them won't make a difference.

I have no issue saying how things are, and this angers people. I think this frustrates them to think someone could have no filter in many specific situations. For example, when someone asks a question about children and so on, I never say 'my son passed away'. I state it as is, 'my son died' (while in the womb at seven months). I refuse to sugar coat things because people refuse to see the world for what it is. This specific situation doesn't anger people, but makes them feel bad. It should.

I will tell the truth, even though somebody else may become offended by those words. None of what I say is truly negative. Although many will internalize how I say something to mean I am callous or without feeling.

All of this could not be further from the truth. I verbally communicate in a way that leaves no room for a pointless back and forth. There are exceptions of course, but that is normally with my wife. If there is one person I try not to offend, it would be my wife. I fail and will continue to do so, but it's the thought that counts!

At the end of it all if anything, I am the one who has to deal with people. Not the other way around. Since so many people believe I should do certain things like from eating with a fork to speaking in a non-black-and-white manner, they believe they have the right to correct what I do or how I say things. I know it should be obvious, but don't ever do that! To state it plainly, that's just rude and obnoxious.

Many people will never get used to that, but others like my wife, must adapt. The easiest example of this was when she'd say something, and I replied with 'interesting'. For a long time, she would get offended and thought 'clearly, there must be subtext to that!' She would further inquire, and she'd get her feelings hurt when I would reply 'it means what you said is interesting. I don't think I could make it any clearer'. I would think the only needed use of subtext is if you're flirting with someone.

I know it's been hard for her to adjust to the way I see the world. The reality is that my normal is a logic based normal. I'm aware I can be unclear at times, but that's usually when I'm speaking with my wife or family. Otherwise, the reason I do or say things is based through logic. Often times, others don't base their normal on a logic based normal.

I've never understood why this is something that is so commonplace.

I don't see the value of playing games with people, as it benefits no one. I feel that most of the world plays this game of political intrigue everywhere around the globe, and I'll never understand that. Instead of stating how things are, people use a cloak of deceit to hide their real intentions. I have lost several friends due to this, because I would NOT abide by their racist outlooks.

When you look at Quebec with their new Loi 21 (Law 21), or if you look at France. Both have laws which clearly discriminate against Muslimas and Jewish women, as we well as against Sikh men (Quebec only as far as I know for Sikh men). I will never understand how or why things like hijabs, burqas, niqabs or turbans would be banned. This is NOT a security risk in any way, shape or form. It's simple crystal-clear racism, because apparently colonialism wasn't enough to subjugate the rest of the globe. Some of their descendants had to do the same, just because of white privilege, and because they feel uncomfortable with diversity.

People play games and deny it, and say they're an open society. No, it's not, and I am ashamed of living where I live because of this. See, black and white. This is so crystal-clear, that it baffles me when I see the rest of the world partake in such erratic behaviour. I've had to adjust to the rest of the world, and that has been a nightmare.

The way I envision the world is one where we can all get along, regardless of gender, colour, language or religion. I don't mind the occasional petty squabbles. But, not when it comes to human rights. Having to adjust to seeing a veil of deceit, while seeing right through it, baffles me. I have to spend energy avoiding that constant barrage of hate, fearmongering and disdain for human life. I do what I can, but I'm still only one man.

At the end of the day, this is why I see myself as typical, and the rest as atypical. To hate is abnormal. To fear is abnormal. To create excuses for racism is a cowardly act born from both white privilege and racism.

Why does logic have to be a rare commodity instead of something which makes sense? Dealing with others can be tiring at times, as my view is fairly simple. I strongly believe that those of us considered outliers (even though we're not) have the most logical approach to life.

If you're unaware of the singer Scatman John, I suggest you listen to his songs. He died in nineteen ninety-nine, but he was ahead of his time with his songs. They were about living together, peace and full acceptance of other human beings. I consider him to be the only singer that ever truly cared about people.

When I see people like him in the public eye state what he did without fear, it gives me hope to a certain degree. I know I'll never be him nor replace him, but I do believe there is hope because of him and others like him. This is the world I want to see.

Through this journey, which is life, Earth is but a stop. This veil of deceit forged by this world is the quickest way off the path to Jannah (Heaven). The more hate is fed, the more you wander off the path to Jannah. The penultimate height for humanity is to reach for the stars. Though, if you stack acts of hatred on top of each other, then we as giants, fall. And when we descend from grace, the harder the fall.

If we remember that we are simple creatures, fashioned somewhere down the line, perhaps we can recall how humanity once was. Without a voice, without love, without ingenuity, and without a care in the world. Perhaps we shall then remember that how we wish to be treated is the same as how we should treat others.

We are but grains of sand on a vast earth, and we, as the human race, somehow believe it's ok to treat others like they're worth less than a grain of sand. Until people acknowledge that there is only one race, I fear that we will never get along, nor treat each other the way we should. Maybe those with down syndrome will have known Jannah (Heaven) before any of us, because of their inability to create such a complex web of hatred. Only humans act this way; that says a lot about what we are, more than who we are.

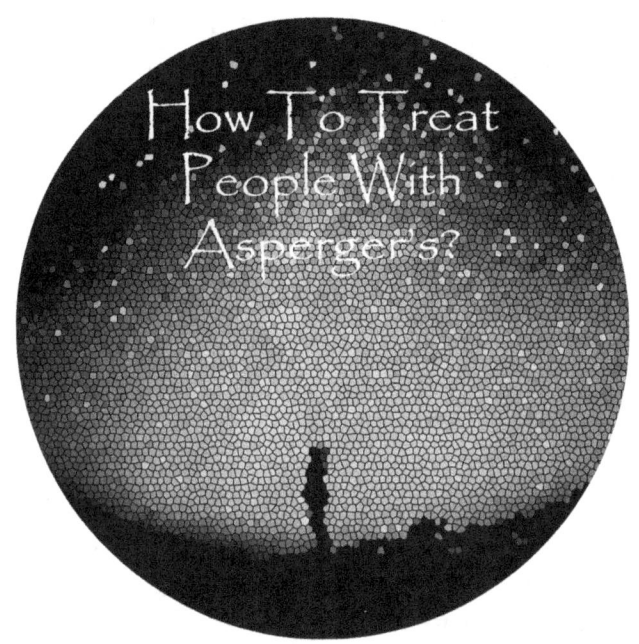

How To Treat People With Aspergers?

The same way you would treat anyone else is how you should treat us. Mostly. Be conscientious of the fact that our behaviour is different in certain aspects. If anything, we can bring a new perspective to your own approach. To assume that one approach is right for everyone is an extremely erroneous and dangerous concept. We, as humans, are different from one another. This is true for anyone. Personally, I have a lot to offer that may compensate for a gap between two opposing views, which can be helpful in supervisory roles or the like.

In terms of non-job related matters, people are different both on a personal level or even on the job, actually. For me, just remember that there are certain things that bother me immensely, and decisions made by others can frustrate me more than it would someone else. If anything, be conscious of that.

This impacts how I react to certain stimuli. I would definitely be the last choice for you if you needed someone at massive events with lots of people in proximity, as I don't deal well with large crowds. The same is true concerning other situations as well.

I remember my wife and I once went to a concert-like event. At the time, neither my wife nor I knew I had Asperger's. The music was much too loud for me, that I literally had to put my fingers in my ears to drown out the noise. Obviously not the most ideal situation. Ultimately, I left. I know my wife was frustrated with the situation, but I didn't know how to explain to her how I felt.

The reality is that loud music or loud noise is not something I can deal with very well. It bothers me to an extreme degree. I have never gone to a concert, and never will for that reason. If anything, I need to get as far away as possible from loud music or loud noises. There may be other stimuli that either bother me or someone else to that type of degree.

Since I am an extremely physically sensitive person, it can get quite difficult for me to deal with wearing certain type of clothes. Especially if not tailored or slightly too small, as I keep rearranging my t-shirt (as often, that is the piece of clothing that always feels slightly too small). Aside from what others consider annoyances, these forms of stimuli can be quite irritating or outright unbearable.

I wouldn't expect a neurotypical person to understand, as these are things they never have to deal with. Try explaining to someone else why walking over the cement cracks on a sidewalk has to be done. I mean, it doesn't make much sense, but I do understand where those people are coming from.

As for 'treating' the person I am, I can do certain things that most people are not very good at. Which means if you need a different perspective, a computer expert, an editor or a creative writer, I would be that person that could accomplish something inhouse instead of you searching for someone who only specializes in that.

The reality is that people like me can specialize in multiple things. I am both a computer expert and a published author. Most individuals would have to only specialize in a single focus. This is fine, but at least, I can accomplish multiple tasks that otherwise would require a second person to help with the project. Furthermore, because I never went to school for these specifically, that is a tremendous advantage. It allowed me to go to university and study more in depth two subjects I wanted to know more about – history and religions (specifically Islam).

hen I went to professional school for web t allowed me to learn the basics for web nd programming. That being said, and just to be clear, I don't specialize in that. Rather, I specialize in Windows and hardware related matters – which is not something I learnt at school – which is extremely different from web design (just to be crystal clear, no I do not have a certificate in anything Windows related). At least, web design has allowed me to have an understanding I would otherwise never had, and it has served me a lot. Especially when it comes to utilizing software like Photoshop or InDesign from Adobe.

Despite not specializing in the software and website aspects in my line of work, it has greatly improved my understanding of technology, while adding to my expertise with computer hardware. Additionally, it has aided me to understand the security aspect of protecting my computer correctly. This has added a layer of understanding to what I can do.

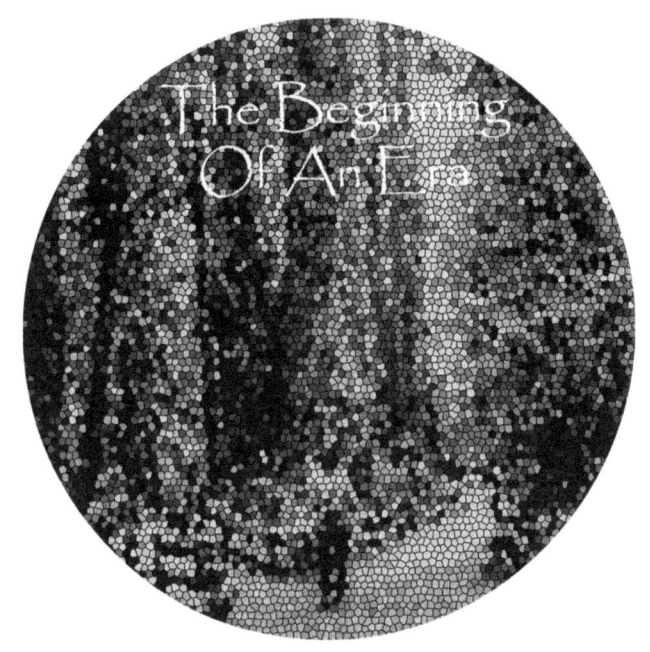

The Beginning Of An Era

The saying goes as such: 'Ignorance is bliss'. Is it, or is it just an excuse to overlook serious matters? It depends on the situation, and the reasoning behind it. When it comes to Asperger's, not knowing can be a painful experience over the stretch of several decades. When you finally understand that the person you are has a basis behind a reasonable explanation, it allows you to comprehend why you are the individual you are.

All those years of people judging you because your best friend is your videogame console, or that you prefer the indoors instead of the loud, obnoxious crowds, or even the older music and movies as you live in a past that still exists for you, it all makes sense. It dawns on you that you couldn't be different than who you are, and you wouldn't want to anyhow. The nineties for the win!

The fact that you are better at a single thing (or two), allows you to understand why you're better than someone else in those specific areas. At the end of it all, you have a better grasp on these, and they seem so seamless to you, that you have no answer as to why you're very good at those.

People keep (annoyingly) asking you: 'You did that?' To which you would answer 'No, I hired a flawless AI from the future'. You obviously have never said that to anyone, but it feels like the perfect answer. It often feels that some people can't believe you're great at something, because you seem different than them somehow. That moment you realise that you have the ability to focus on something, you keep at it.

That instant where your craft has the ability to make others laugh, cry or think more profoundly about life, you know you're doing something special. Finally, when you get to fathom why you have that or those abilities, it starts making sense. The next step is to share it, in the hopes that people take notice and talk about it to others, so it can be shared with as many individuals as possible.

Ultimately, what seems like petty annoyances at best to most, there is a reason as to why it feels like the world is crumbling around you. Depending on the person you are, that could be meltdowns altogether, seemingly everlasting frustrations or even an irritating sense of being. Regardless of those you may or may not have, there is a relief understanding there is a reason for any of those to occur.

I personally don't have meltdowns, but for those who do, they at that point understand why. As for the rest, having an explanation that makes sense, it feels good knowing that it's not because you're just hypersensitive or anything. I mean, you are, but it's because there's a rational explanation behind it. No more nights wondering why. Although, there might be many sleepless ones or half-sleeps that tire you out due to your anxiety.

Sure, many people still don't understand why you do the things you do, and frankly, it's none of their business. You owe nothing to anyone. After all, I have met extremely frustrating and aggravating people, and I don't ever wonder why. It could be because they have Asperger's, a bad upbringing, or they're simply obnoxious. There isn't always a rational explanation, sometimes people are just selfish.

There are times where I appeared as annoying or obnoxious to some people, including family, but at least there is a valid reason behind it. It wasn't because I was doing anything on purpose. As my cousin, trying to spare my feelings once, as I asked if I was annoying, he said after a few deliberate seconds of thinking: 'You're persistent'. Yeah... short of an insult to be sure. But I appreciate his thoughtful, carefully chosen words, nonetheless.

All in all, the way I am may be why I avoid trying to make new friends at this point. I just know that those who've stopped speaking to me for X reason never bothered to tell me why they stopped talking to me. I consider that to be beyond contemptuous, as well as extremely insulting. I certainly don't need that type of childish behaviour in my life. So, I am grateful that they have exited my life. I might not always be easy to be around at times, but it doesn't mean I need to settle for being with those who think they are better than me.

For better or worse, like anyone else, I can be extraordinary or frustrating to be around. If anything, I bring a boatload of creativity to the table. Whether or not people want to acknowledge that is up to them. Regardless, the way I see the world is certainly amazing, as my approach is fairly different. Thinking outside the box you say? Who needs a box?!

I want the world to be my canvas, as I create a new world through writing and music. The journey itself in this world is merely a step towards a new life down the road. Be it in fifty or a hundred years from now. Whatever mark I leave on it may not matter much in the grand scheme of things, yet it allows my soul to expand beyond who and what I am.

While the world sees this universe as linear, I don't. As others see Earth as a small world, I see it as a millionth of a grain of sand within a millionth of a galaxy. Finally, when individuals see their potential as infinitely finite (a true paradox!), I see my potential as only limited by my self-impositions.

My life is both a curse and a blessing, but I wouldn't trade the person I am for anything in the world. All I can ever see as I look unto others, is what they decide to show the rest of us. Their lives may be amazing, just as much as they could be horrendous. For better or worse, I would prefer the certainty that I know to be my life.

In the end, I am who I am. For all those I have made happy, sad, frustrated and/or annoyed, those parts of me aren't going anywhere. I shall remain the man that I am until I am no more in this world. If anything, Asperger's has not defined who I am, it is who I am. It is not a part of me, as I can't separate the person I am with how I am. The way my brain is wired is the way it is for whatever reason it decided to wire itself.